<u>Simple explanation</u>

<u>Of</u>

<u>Mental problems</u>

<u>Preface</u>

Dear readers,

I wrote this book to give you a clear understanding of the world of mental health in everyday language. It's meant to encourage you to engage with the topic and find solutions to your own challenges.

Mental health issues affect all of us in different ways. Whether you're personally affected or know someone who needs help, you're not alone. In this book, you'll find information and practical tips to help you better understand how mental health problems arise and how to cope with them.

I invite you to continue reading with an open heart and a curious mind. We can only overcome the stigma surrounding mental health issues through knowledge and understanding. My hope is that this book will help you find confidence in your own strength and discover paths to healing.

Warm regards,

Kevin van Olafson

<u>Chapter 1: Introduction</u>

Chapter 1: Introduction

In the first chapter of this book, I provide an overview of the book and its objectives. The book focuses on the topic of mental health issues and aims to help you develop a better understanding of your own mental well-being.

Mental health issues are something many people around the world struggle with. They can have various impacts on our lives, affecting our relationships, daily routines, and overall well-being. The book covers different mental health topics such as depression, anxiety disorders, eating disorders, addiction disorders, and much more.

In the introduction, the fundamental question is addressed: What are mental health issues exactly? I provide a precise definition and explain that mental health problems can be influenced by various factors. These include genetic predispositions, biological factors such as imbalances in brain neurotransmitters, and environmental factors such as traumatic experiences or stress.

I also give a preview of the upcoming chapters and explain which aspects will be covered to provide a comprehensive understanding of mental health issues. It's important for me to emphasize that my book is not intended as a substitute for professional help or medical advice but rather as an information source and guide for individuals who want to better understand their own mental health and learn about possible sources of assistance.

I conclude the introduction by encouraging open discussions about mental health issues and seeking support. There is hope and healing, and my book aims to provide you with tools and information to pave the way towards improved mental well-being.

"This first chapter serves as an introduction to the topic, preparing you for the subsequent chapters where we will delve deeper into specific mental health issues. I want to provide you with a foundation for understanding mental health and encourage you to explore your own mental state and seek help if needed."

Chapter 2: What Are Mental Health Issues?

Mental health issues are conditions that affect our emotional and mental well-being. They influence our thoughts, feelings, and behaviors in various ways.

Mental health issues can range from milder challenges to more severe disorders and impact different aspects of our lives.

Defining mental health issues precisely is not always easy since they encompass a broad spectrum of conditions. However, there are common characteristics that characterize them. Mental health issues can manifest through persistent negative emotions such as sadness, anxiety, or anger. They can also lead to isolating ourselves, struggling with daily functioning, or affecting our overall quality of life.

It's important to understand that mental health issues are not due to a lack of strength or willpower. They are medical conditions that can be influenced by various factors. Genetic predispositions, imbalances in brain neurotransmitters, traumatic experiences, chronic stress, or certain life circumstances can contribute to mental health problems.

Mental health issues can take various forms, such as anxiety disorders, depression, eating disorders, addiction disorders, or personality disorders. In my book, I will delve into these specific problems in more detail and provide a thorough explanation of their characteristics, causes, and treatment options.

It's crucial to emphasize that mental health issues are common, and seeking help is not something to be ashamed of. By educating ourselves about mental health issues and talking about them, we can reduce stigma and improve support for those affected.

"This chapter aims to provide you with a more comprehensive definition and a clearer overview of mental health issues. My goal is to help you develop a better understanding of these conditions and realize that you are not alone in your experiences. In the following chapters, I will delve into specific mental health issues in more detail and present various treatment and support options."

<u>Chapter 3: The Role of Genetics</u>

Genetics play a significant role in passing traits from one generation to another. Our genes contain information that determines how our bodies are built and how they function. It is also known that certain genes can be associated with an increased risk of mental health issues.

Studies have shown that there are specific genetic factors that can increase the risk of mental health problems. If we have a family history of mental disorders, we may have a higher risk of developing similar issues. However, this doesn't mean that we will automatically have mental health problems, as other factors also come into play.

It's important to note that genetics is not the sole factor that determines our mental health. Environmental factors also play a crucial role. Certain genes may increase the risk of mental health problems, but it is in combination with specific environmental factors like traumatic experiences or chronic stress that problems may arise.

Genetics can also explain why certain individuals may be more susceptible to specific mental health issues than others. For example, there are certain genes associated with an increased risk of depression or anxiety disorders. However, this doesn't mean that a person will inevitably develop these problems. It is a complex interplay of genetics, environmental factors, and individual life experiences.

It's important to emphasize that genetic predisposition is just one piece of the puzzle. It doesn't mean that we have no control over our mental health. There are various ways we can strengthen our mental well-being regardless of our genetic predispositions. These include healthy lifestyle habits, social support, stress management techniques, and seeking professional help if needed.

In addition to the inheritance of genes, there are also epigenetic factors that can influence our mental health. Epigenetics refers to changes in gene expression that are not due to changes in the DNA sequence itself.

These epigenetic changes can be triggered by environmental factors and can lead to the activation or deactivation of certain genes.

Studies have shown that environmental factors such as stress, diet, lifestyle, and traumatic experiences can induce epigenetic changes that may increase or decrease the risk of mental health issues. These findings highlight the interconnection between genetics and the environment, and how their interaction plays a crucial role in the development of mental health problems.

Another important aspect is the examination of resilience and protective factors. Despite genetic predispositions or challenging environmental factors, people can possess resilient traits that strengthen their mental health and make them more resistant to mental health problems.

Such protective factors can include a supportive family, positive social support, healthy coping strategies, and a stable environment.

It's also important to note that genetics and epigenetic factors are not static. Studies have shown that our lifestyle and environment can also influence our genes. Healthy behaviors such as regular exercise, balanced diet, and sufficient sleep can bring about genetic changes that contribute to better mental health.

"Overall, the third chapter emphasizes that the role of genetics in mental health problems is complex and influenced by various factors. Our genes may bring an increased risk of mental health issues, but it's important to understand that it is not our destiny. By better understanding the genetic and epigenetic connections, promoting healthy habits, and accessing appropriate support, we can positively influence our mental well-being."

Chapter 4: Biological Foundations of Mental Health Problems

Neurotransmitters are like little chemical messengers in the brain that are responsible for transmitting information between nerve cells. If there's something off or out of balance with these neurotransmitters, it can lead to mental disorders.

At the beginning of the chapter, we introduce the basic neurotransmitters that play an important role in psychology. One of the most well-known neurotransmitters is serotonin, which is involved in regulating mood, sleep, appetite, and pain perception. When there's an imbalance in the availability or uptake of serotonin in the brain, it can lead to depression and anxiety disorders. Another important neurotransmitter is dopamine, which is associated with reward, motivation, and movement coordination. An imbalance in dopamine function can result in disorders like Parkinson's disease or schizophrenia.

Besides serotonin and dopamine, other neurotransmitters also play a crucial role in regulating mental health. Noradrenaline influences attention, responsiveness, and mood, while GABA (Gamma-Aminobutyric Acid) has a calming effect and reduces anxiety.

Glutamate is the brain's primary excitatory neurotransmitter and is involved in learning, memory formation, and neural plasticity.

We also explain how neurotransmitters work in the brain. When one nerve cell sends a signal to another nerve cell, it releases neurotransmitters that bind to receptors on the surface of the target cell. This binding triggers a reaction in the target cell, allowing the signal to be transmitted. An imbalance in neurotransmitters can disrupt signal transmission and lead to malfunctions in the brain.

Another important aspect we address is the significance of brain chemistry in mental disorders. The brain is a highly complex organ where numerous chemical processes take place. Brain chemistry encompasses the composition and activity of various neurotransmitters, enzymes, hormones, and other molecules in the brain. An anomaly in brain chemistry can affect the function and communication of nerve cells, thus causing mental disorders.

We also examine the influence of genetics and environmental factors on brain chemistry and the development of mental problems. Genetic factors can influence the production, breakdown, or receptors of neurotransmitters, increasing the risk of mental disorders. Environmental factors such as stress, traumatic experiences, or substance abuse can also impact brain chemistry and raise the risk of mental problems.

Later in the chapter, we explore various mental disorders in relation to their biological foundations. We investigate how dysregulation of neurotransmitters and brain chemistry can play a role in disorders such as depression, anxiety disorders, eating disorders, substance use disorders, and post-traumatic stress disorder (PTSD). We explain which specific neurotransmitter systems may be affected and how this influences symptoms and treatment options.

It's important to note that the biological foundations of mental health problems are very complex, and mental disorders are not solely attributed to biological factors. They often arise from a combination of biological, psychological, and social factors. Nonetheless, understanding neurochemical processes and the role of neurotransmitters in the brain provides valuable insights into the origins and treatment of mental problems.

"Overall, this chapter highlights the complex connection between brain chemistry and mental health. It emphasizes the importance of a balanced neurotransmitter system and healthy brain function for psychological well-being. Understanding these biological foundations can aid in better comprehending mental disorders and developing targeted treatment approaches."

Chapter 5: Influence of Environmental Factors on Mental Health

Our life circumstances and the environment we live in play a crucial role in our well-being. Different environmental factors can have both positive and negative effects on our mental health, so it's important to carefully consider them.

One key environmental factor is social connection. Having a supportive family, close friendships, and a strong social network can give us a sense of appreciation and belonging. This boosts our self-esteem and helps us better cope with stress and challenges.

Positive interpersonal relationships can provide us with emotional support, comfort, and practical help during difficult times.

On the other hand, social isolation, loneliness, bullying, or ongoing relationship conflicts can have negative effects on our mental health and increase the risk of mental problems.

The quality of our childhood and adolescence also plays a crucial role. Experiences during early life stages can have long-term effects on our mental health. Childhood traumas such as abuse, neglect, or traumatic events can lead to lasting emotional and psychological distress. These can affect our coping abilities, self-confidence, and interpersonal relationships, thereby increasing the risk of mental problems in adulthood.

However, it's important to emphasize that healing, therapy, and support in coping with traumatic experiences are possible.

Another significant environmental factor that influences our mental health is the workplace. A healthy work environment that provides support, recognition, and appropriate working conditions can contribute to positive mental health. Achieving a work-life balance, having adequate breaks, a respectful work atmosphere, and the opportunity to utilize skills and talents can promote well-being in the workplace.

Conversely, stress, overwork, bullying, conflicts, or a lack of job satisfaction can lead to mental problems. It's important to pay attention to our own needs and, if necessary, take steps to create a healthy work environment or seek support in managing workplace stress.

Access to education, healthcare, and social resources also plays a significant role in mental health. Education enables us to acquire skills and knowledge that help us cope with life's challenges. Individuals with better educational opportunities often have more resources and strategies to promote their mental health and cope with mental problems.

Access to adequate healthcare is also crucial. Comprehensive medical care, including mental health services, can enable the detection, treatment, and support of mental problems.

Lack of access to such services can result in undetected and worsening mental problems. Therefore, it's important for healthcare systems to provide appropriate resources for mental health and eliminate barriers to ensure comprehensive care for all.

Furthermore, ecological factors can also influence our mental health. A healthy and clean environment, access to green spaces and nature, a safe neighborhood, and adequate infrastructure contribute to our well-being. An environment that offers safety, tranquility, and relaxation can reduce stress and promote mental health.

It's important to note that environmental factors are not always within our control, and we may not always have the ability to change our circumstances. In such cases, it's crucial to seek support and develop coping strategies to deal with the challenges. This may involve seeking social support, learning healthy coping mechanisms, or seeking professional help.

"All in all, this fifth chapter highlights how various environmental factors can influence our mental health. It emphasizes the importance of a supportive social environment, a healthy childhood, a positive workplace, good access to education and healthcare, and a pleasant ecological environment. By considering these factors, we can better understand our mental health and take targeted actions to promote it and address mental problems. The next chapter will focus on proven strategies and techniques to cope with our environmental factors and strengthen our mental health."

Chapter 6: Types of Mental Disorders

In this chapter, we'll cover different categories of mental disorders that are frequently diagnosed and have a significant impact on the lives of those affected. It's crucial to understand the diversity of these disorders in order to raise awareness and potentially assist individuals who may be affected.

One significant category of mental disorders is anxiety disorders. These are characterized by persistent and excessive fears and worries. An example of an anxiety disorder is generalized anxiety disorder, where a person experiences chronic and excessive worry even when there is no specific threat.

Another form of anxiety disorder is panic disorder, which involves recurring and unpredictable panic attacks. Other types of anxiety disorders include social phobia, which entails intense fears in social situations, and specific phobias, where there is an excessive fear of certain objects or situations.

Agoraphobia, on the other hand, refers to the fear of public places or situations where escape might be difficult.

Mood disorders are another significant category of mental illnesses. They affect emotional states and can significantly impair daily life. The most well-known mood disorder is depression, where a person feels consistently down for an extended period, loses interest in activities, experiences decreased energy, and exhibits negative thought patterns. Another common mood disorder is bipolar disorder, characterized by episodic phases of depression and mania.

During a depressive phase, the affected person feels similar to depression, while manic phases involve elevated mood, increased energy, and impulsive behavior.

Personality disorders are deeply ingrained and long-lasting patterns of thinking, feeling, and behavior that deviate from the norm and cause significant functional impairments. Borderline personality disorder is a frequently diagnosed personality disorder, marked by unstable relationships, impulsivity, identity uncertainty, and intense mood swings. Narcissistic personality disorder, on the other hand, manifests as an excessive need for admiration, inflated self-esteem, and a lack of empathy. Antisocial personality disorder is characterized by repeated misconduct, disregard for others' rights, and a lack of empathy.

Another relevant area of mental disorders is eating disorders, which involve eating behavior and body perception. Anorexia nervosa is an eating disorder characterized by severely restricted food intake and an intense desire to be thin. Conversely, individuals with bulimia experience repeated episodes of binge eating followed by compensatory behaviors like vomiting or excessive exercise. Binge-eating disorder involves regular episodes of binge eating but without compensatory measures.

Substance use disorders are also of great importance as they can significantly impair quality of life. Alcohol and drug addiction are well-known examples of substance use disorders. People with substance abuse problems have a compulsive craving for substances and cannot control their behavior, leading to severe health, social, and occupational consequences.

In addition to substance dependencies, gambling addiction can also be considered a form of addiction where individuals have an uncontrollable urge to gamble and continue despite negative consequences.

Post-traumatic stress disorder (PTSD) is another important mental disorder. It occurs as a reaction to a traumatic event that has left a deep emotional wound. People with PTSD experience recurring traumatic memories, nightmares, excessive tension, and avoidance behavior. Coping with PTSD often requires professional support and can be a long-term challenge.

In the context of the workplace, mental health problems also play a significant role. Stress, burnout, and bullying are just a few of the challenges employees may face. Workplace stressors can negatively affect mental health and contribute to various disorders.

Treatment options for mental disorders encompass various approaches. Psychotherapy is a common method where a therapeutic relationship is established to help individuals understand and cope with their problems.

Medication may also play a role, especially in severe cases where pharmacological support is necessary. Additionally, alternative approaches like relaxation techniques, physical activity, and complementary therapy methods can be used alongside conventional treatment.

Dealing with mental problems in everyday life is another important aspect. Self-care, stress management techniques, and seeking support in social circles are crucial for maintaining mental health. Sharing experiences with other affected individuals, learning stress management strategies, and creating a supportive environment can help manage mental problems and promote the healing process.

Lastly, the book also provides stories of individuals who have successfully overcome their mental problems. These stories serve as a source of hope and demonstrate that it is possible to cope with mental disorders and find healing. They emphasize that support, treatment, and self-care are crucial factors in regaining mental health and leading a fulfilling life.

"This chapter provides a comprehensive overview of the different types of mental disorders. It's important to emphasize that an accurate diagnosis and treatment should be sought from professionals in the field of mental health, as

they possess the necessary expertise and experience to offer appropriate support and treatment."

Chapter 7: Depression: Causes, Symptoms, and Treatment Options

When I delved into the topic of depression, I was amazed by how complex this condition is and the impact it can have on the lives of those affected. In this chapter, I want to give you a comprehensive insight into the causes, symptoms, and treatment options for depression.

Causes of Depression:
It's important to understand that depression is not caused by a single factor but rather a combination of various factors. Genetic predisposition can play a role, which means the risk of depression may be higher in families. However, it doesn't mean that depression is inevitably inherited; rather, genetic predisposition is one possible factor. Additionally, biochemical imbalances in the brain, particularly involving the neurotransmitters serotonin, norepinephrine, and dopamine, may be involved in the development of depression. These neurotransmitters play a crucial role in regulating mood and emotions, and disturbances in their balance can lead to depressive symptoms.

Environmental factors such as traumatic events, chronic stress, loss, and social isolation can also increase the risk of depression. Understanding these different factors is important for gaining a holistic understanding of the condition and finding appropriate treatment approaches.

Symptoms of Depression:
Depression is not only manifested in emotional symptoms such as persistent sadness, hopelessness, and loss of interest but also in physical symptoms such as fatigue, sleep disturbances, appetite changes, and bodily discomfort. Moreover, cognitive symptoms such as concentration and memory problems can occur, and individuals with depression often have negative thoughts and feelings of worthlessness and guilt. It's important to recognize that these symptoms should be taken seriously and not simply ignored. They often lead

to significant impairments in daily life and affect the quality of life of those affected. Therefore, it is of great importance to recognize the symptoms and seek professional help.

<u>Treatment Options:</u>
There are various approaches to treating depression, and it's important to emphasize that not every treatment method is equally effective for everyone. One of the most common and effective treatment methods is psychotherapy, particularly cognitive-behavioral therapy (CBT). This therapy aims to identify and change negative thinking patterns while developing healthy behavioral patterns.

In some cases, medication treatment in the form of antidepressants may be recommended to regulate the biochemical balance in the brain. It's important to take these medications under medical supervision and be aware of possible side effects. In addition to traditional therapy, there are also alternative approaches such as sports therapy, art therapy, and relaxation techniques that can be supportive. Each person is unique, so it's important to find an individualized approach that best suits their needs and preferences.

In conclusion, I want to emphasize that depression is a serious condition that should not be faced alone. It takes courage to seek help and accept support. Professional therapists, psychiatrists, and support groups can assist in the journey to recovery. At the same time, I want to encourage you and emphasize that there is hope and healing.

"In this chapter, we explored the causes, symptoms, and treatment options for depression to develop a better understanding of this condition. I hope this information will help you and other individuals affected by depression to find the right path to recovery and seek support for leading a fulfilling and happy life."

<u>Chapter 8: Anxiety Disorders</u>

In the chapter on "Anxiety Disorders," we discuss various types of mental disorders characterized by excessive and persistent fears. Anxiety is a normal body reaction to potential threats, but for people with anxiety disorders, this natural sense of fear spirals out of control and significantly impairs their daily lives.

One common form of anxiety disorder is generalized anxiety disorder (GAD). People with GAD experience chronic and excessive worry and anxiety about various areas of life, even when there are no specific or obvious reasons for concern. They constantly worry about everyday things like work, finances, health, or interpersonal relationships. This constant worry leads to persistent tension, sleep disturbances, difficulties with concentration, and physical symptoms such as muscle tension or headaches.

Another type of anxiety disorder is panic disorder. People with panic disorder suffer from recurrent and sudden panic attacks that occur unexpectedly and are accompanied by intense fear. During a panic attack, physical symptoms such as rapid heart rate, shortness of breath, dizziness, and a sense of losing control can occur. The fear of experiencing further panic attacks can lead individuals to avoid certain places or situations, a condition known as agoraphobia.

Social phobia is another form of anxiety disorder in which people have overwhelming fear of social situations. They feel anxious and uncomfortable in the presence of others, fear being observed or evaluated, and therefore avoid social interactions. This fear can greatly impact personal and professional life, leading to isolation.

In addition to these three main types of anxiety disorders, there are also specific phobias. These involve irrational and excessive fear of certain objects or situations such as spiders, heights, flying, or confined spaces. People with specific phobias often experience a strong urge to avoid these triggers to prevent the associated anxiety.

It's important to note that anxiety disorders are treatable. Treatment typically involves a combination of psychotherapy and, if necessary, medication support. Cognitive-behavioral therapy (CBT) is a commonly used therapeutic approach that identifies and modifies negative thought patterns and behavioral patterns contributing to anxiety. In some cases, medications such as selective serotonin reuptake inhibitors (SSRIs) or benzodiazepines may be prescribed to alleviate symptoms.

"Understanding the different types of anxiety disorders can help raise awareness of these conditions and assist individuals in seeking support and appropriate treatment. By being aware of the symptoms and knowing that help is available, we can contribute to reducing the stigma associated with anxiety disorders and pave the way for better mental health."

Chapter 9: Eating Disorders

In the chapter on "Eating Disorders," we discuss various disorders that affect eating behavior and body perception. Eating disorders are serious mental illnesses that can have both physical and emotional consequences.

One of the most well-known eating disorders is anorexia, also known as anorexia nervosa. People with this disorder have a strong fear of weight gain and a distorted body perception, perceiving themselves as overweight even when they are actually severely underweight.

Individuals with anorexia often adhere to strict diets, severely restrict their food intake, and engage in excessive physical activities to lose weight. This behavior can lead to significant health problems such as nutrient deficiencies, muscle wasting, osteoporosis, and heart issues.

Another eating disorder is bulimia. Individuals with bulimia experience recurrent episodes of binge eating, where they consume large amounts of food in a short period of time. However, after these binge episodes, they feel overwhelming shame and guilt. To control their weight or prevent weight gain, they engage in compensatory measures such as vomiting, excessive exercise, or the misuse of laxatives or diuretics.

Bulimia can lead to serious health problems such as dental issues, electrolyte imbalances, gastrointestinal problems, and heart rhythm disturbances.

Binge-eating disorder is another form of eating disorder in which individuals repeatedly experience binge eating episodes but do not engage in compensatory measures. They feel a loss of control over their eating behavior and consume large amounts of food in a short period of time.

Affected individuals often suffer from intense feelings of shame, guilt, and discomfort due to their eating behavior. Binge-eating disorder can result in weight gain, obesity, diabetes, and other health complications.

Eating disorders can have serious impacts on physical and mental health. They are often caused by a combination of factors, including genetic, biological, psychological, and social influences. Societal beauty ideals, perfectionism, low self-esteem, and traumatic experiences can also play a role.

Treating eating disorders usually requires a comprehensive approach. A combination of psychotherapeutic support, nutritional counseling, and medical care can be employed to help those affected.

The goal is to develop a healthy relationship with food, positive body perception, and emotional well-being. Early intervention is important to achieve the best results and avoid potential complications.

"It is important to emphasize that eating disorders are serious illnesses that require professional help. If you or someone you know shows signs of an eating disorder, it is important to seek support from mental health professionals. Help is available, and with proper treatment and support, individuals with eating disorders can find their way to a healthy relationship with food and themselves."

Chapter 10: Addiction

This chapter focuses on the problematic use of substances like alcohol, drugs, and gambling. Addiction is a complex mental disorder that can cause both physical and psychological dependency.

For me personally, the topic of addiction is of great importance as I've had close friends or family members who struggled with the effects of addiction. It's important to understand that addiction can affect people from all walks of life and is not due to a lack of willpower or character weakness. Rather, it's a complex illness influenced by a combination of genetic, biological, psychological, and environmental factors.

The misuse of substances like alcohol, drugs, and excessive gambling can initially serve as a form of relief or coping mechanism for stress, trauma, or emotional difficulties. People may use them as an escape to avoid problems or numb negative feelings.

However, over time, this can develop into a dependency where the consumption of the substance or the act of gambling becomes compulsive and negatively impacts the individual's life.

Addiction can have various consequences. Physically, it can lead to health problems such as liver damage, cardiovascular diseases, lung issues, and infectious diseases. Substance dependence can also cause withdrawal symptoms when the body tries to adapt to the absence of the substance.

Psychologically, anxiety, depression, paranoia, and impaired judgment can develop. Social consequences such as the loss of friendships, family conflicts, financial problems, and job loss can also occur.

It's important to understand that addiction can be treated. The first step is acknowledging the problem and seeking professional help. Treatment often involves a combination of medical care, therapy, and social support.

Detoxification, rehabilitation programs, and withdrawal therapies can help manage the withdrawal process and overcome physical dependence. Therapy approaches like cognitive-behavioral therapy, motivational interviews, and support groups can help address psychological dependency and learn new coping strategies.

For individuals and their loved ones, receiving support and understanding is crucial. Good social support can have a positive impact on the recovery process. However, it's also important to emphasize that the path to recovery is often a long and challenging one that may involve relapses. Nevertheless, it is possible to live a life free from addiction and bring about positive change.

"I hope this more detailed explanation provides you with a deeper understanding of the topic of addiction and highlights the importance of support and treatment for individuals and their loved ones. If you or someone you know is struggling with addiction, I encourage you to seek professional help and accept support."

Chapter 11: Post-Traumatic Stress Disorder (PTSD)

Post-Traumatic Stress Disorder (PTSD) is a complex and deep-seated mental illness that can occur after experiencing or witnessing a traumatic event.

Imagine being involved in a situation of extreme danger or threat where your life or the lives of others are at stake. Such events can leave a deep emotional wound and profoundly affect the lives of those involved in various ways.

People with PTSD can experience a wide range of symptoms that significantly impair their daily lives. One of the most noticeable symptoms is recurring and distressing flashbacks, where the affected person relives the traumatic event in all its painful details repeatedly. These flashbacks can occur unexpectedly and transport the person back to the past, causing them to lose control over their present reality.

In addition to flashbacks, distressing nightmares can occur, disrupting sleep and hindering recovery. These nightmares can be so vivid and intense that they fill the person with fear and terror, reawakening the fears and emotions of the trauma. Individuals may also exhibit strong avoidance reactions, avoiding specific places, people, activities, or even conversations that might remind them of the traumatic event. While these avoidance mechanisms serve to reduce pain and distress, they can lead to social isolation and a restricted life.

People with PTSD can also experience negative changes in mood and thinking. They may feel emotionally numb or detached, as if cut off from their own feelings. The world may appear gray and threatening, and they may struggle to experience positive emotions. Furthermore, negative thoughts and beliefs about themselves, others, and the world may prevail. They may feel guilty for not preventing the event or blame themselves for the trauma.

Another common symptom of PTSD is increased arousal, which can manifest in various ways. People with PTSD may be easily irritable, and their patience and tolerance thresholds are often lower than before. They may have difficulties concentrating and maintaining attention. Sleep disturbances are also common, including insomnia, nightmares, or intrusive thoughts that disrupt sleep and lead to fatigue and exhaustion. Additionally, they may display startle reactions, where they startle or overreact to minor triggers.

PTSD can significantly impact the lives of those affected and pose significant challenges. Fortunately, there are effective treatment options for PTSD. Early diagnosis and intervention are crucial for successful treatment.

Therapeutic approaches like cognitive-behavioral therapy have proven particularly effective in alleviating PTSD symptoms and helping individuals process the trauma. Another promising therapy method is Eye Movement Desensitization and Reprocessing (EMDR), where individuals process their traumatic memories through eye movements or other forms of bilateral stimulation.

In some cases, medication can also be used to treat PTSD, especially to alleviate symptoms such as anxiety, depression, or sleep disturbances. However, it is important to note that medication alone does not provide a lasting solution and should be used in combination with other therapeutic approaches.

Strong social support is also crucial for individuals with PTSD. Family, friends, and support groups can play a significant role in supporting and encouraging those affected. By offering understanding, compassion, and support, they can help alleviate feelings of isolation and loneliness.

It is important to understand that PTSD is not a weakness or failure but a natural response to exceptionally distressing events. However, the path to healing may require time, patience, and support. Each person is unique, and the healing process can vary individually.

With the right support and treatment, many people with PTSD can make significant progress and achieve a better quality of life.

"I hope this detailed and easily understandable explanation of Post-Traumatic Stress Disorder (PTSD) has helped you better understand the topic. If you or someone you know is affected by PTSD, I encourage you to seek professional help and accept support. There is hope and paths to healing, and no one should have to fight this burden alone."

Chapter 12: Mental Health in the Workplace

Mental health in the workplace is becoming an increasingly important topic in our modern working world. We spend a significant amount of our time at work, and the impact of the work environment on our mental health should not be underestimated.

A positive work environment can promote our mental health and contribute to our well-being, while a negative work environment can lead to stress, burnout, and other mental health problems.

Stress is a common issue in the workplace and can have negative effects on our mental and physical health. High workloads, time pressure, workplace conflicts, and lack of support can lead to chronic stress. This stress can result in exhaustion, anxiety, sleep disorders, and other mental health problems. Therefore, it is important for employers to take measures to reduce workplace stress and promote a healthy work-life balance.

One aspect of mental strain in the workplace is the lack of autonomy and control. When employees feel that they have no decision-making power, cannot shape their work independently, and constantly have to follow instructions, it can lead to feelings of frustration and helplessness.

It is important for employers to provide employees with a certain level of autonomy and freedom in decision-making. By delegating responsibility, allowing employees to shape their workflow, and involving them in decision-making processes, employers can strengthen the sense of control and reduce mental strain.

Another aspect of mental strain in the workplace is the lack of social support. When employees feel isolated and unsupported, it can lead to feelings of loneliness, stress, and overwhelm. A supportive work environment that promotes open communication, teamwork, and mutual support is therefore of great importance.

Employers should take measures to create a positive organizational culture where colleagues support each other, provide feedback, and find solutions together. Promoting team activities, shared breaks, and social events can also help strengthen the sense of belonging and support.

Furthermore, a good way to improve the work climate is the implementation of mentoring programs. Mentoring allows for the exchange of experiences, knowledge, and resources between experienced employees and younger colleagues.

By establishing mentor-mentee relationships, employees can benefit from valuable insights and support, whether it's in career development, coping with challenges, or promoting well-being. Mentoring programs not only facilitate knowledge transfer but also build relationships and trust in the work environment, contributing to a positive and supportive atmosphere.

Promoting mental health in the workplace requires a holistic approach. Employers should take measures to create a positive work environment that supports the physical and mental health of employees. This includes measures such as flexible work schedules, clear communication, adequate breaks and recovery time, opportunities for development, and promoting a healthy lifestyle. Stress management programs, resilience-building initiatives, and mental health awareness can also be of great benefit.

It is important for employers and managers to foster a culture of open communication and understanding, where employees can talk about their mental health without fear of stigma or negative consequences.

Individuals can also take steps to promote their mental health in the workplace. This includes stress management strategies such as regular breaks, physical activity, healthy eating, and sufficient sleep. Setting realistic goals, prioritizing tasks, and creating a balanced work plan can also help reduce stress. Seeking social support, whether through conversations with colleagues, joining support groups, or accessing professional help when needed, is also important.

"Mental health in the workplace should be seen as a shared responsibility among employers, managers, and employees. By creating a healthy work environment, managing stress, and promoting mental health, we can help make work a positive and enriching experience. By supporting mental health in the workplace, we can enhance the well-being and performance of employees and ultimately create a healthier and more successful work culture."

Chapter 13: Treatment Methods

Now, we'll introduce you to various approaches that can be used to cope with mental health issues. It provides a comprehensive overview of different methods and strategies developed to help people improve their mental health and enhance their quality of life.

One of the most well-known and effective forms of treatment is psychotherapy. In psychotherapy, therapists work closely with individuals to identify the underlying causes of their mental health problems and develop suitable coping strategies. One commonly applied form of psychotherapy is cognitive-behavioral therapy.

Here, negative thinking patterns and behaviors are recognized and changed to bring about positive changes in thinking and actions. By building coping skills, promoting self-reflection, and strengthening self-efficacy, individuals can learn to manage their challenges and create positive changes in their lives.

Medication is often used in combination with psychotherapy, especially for more severe forms of mental disorders. Antidepressants, antipsychotics, and anti-anxiety medications are some of the drugs that can be used to alleviate specific symptoms.

It's important to note that the use of medication should always be done under medical supervision to ensure appropriate dosage and monitoring while minimizing potential side effects.

In addition to traditional psychotherapy and medication, there are alternative approaches that can be used as complements or as standalone treatments. Artistic therapies such as music or art therapy allow for the expression of emotions and experiences in creative ways.

Movement therapies like dance or sports therapy can help reduce physical and emotional tension and increase well-being. Relaxation techniques such as meditation, breathing exercises, and yoga can also be effective means to reduce stress and restore inner balance.

Another important aspect of treating mental health problems lies in creating a positive and supportive work climate. Workplace mental stressors such as stress, burnout, and bullying can have significant impacts on mental health. Employers and leaders play a crucial role in taking measures to promote the mental health of employees.

This includes creating a respectful and inclusive work environment that fosters open communication, collaboration, and support. Flexibility in work scheduling and promoting a healthy work-life balance are also important aspects. Furthermore, training and awareness initiatives for leaders and employees can help raise awareness of mental health and improve support options.

"By familiarizing themselves with different treatment possibilities and tailoring them to their individual needs, people can pursue a holistic approach to improving their mental health. The combination of psychotherapy, medication, alternative approaches, and a positive work environment can lead to a comprehensive treatment plan that helps individuals cope with their mental health issues and find hope for healing and a fulfilling life."

Chapter 14: Dealing with Mental Health Issues in Everyday Life

As we approach the end of our book, in this penultimate chapter, I want to provide you with easily understandable tips and encouraging examples on how to support yourself, manage stress, and find the necessary support. Get ready to strengthen your well-being and discover new ways to deal with mental challenges.

Self-care:
Let's start with a crucial topic: self-care. In our hectic daily lives, we often forget to take care of ourselves. But it's of great importance that you take time to look after yourself. Imagine you've had a long, stressful day and feel exhausted. An example of self-care could be consciously taking a break and indulging in an activity that makes you feel good. It could be reading a good book, listening to your favorite music, or enjoying a relaxing cup of tea. By taking this time for yourself, you replenish your energy and strengthen your mental health.

Stress management:
Another important topic is coping with stress. Stress can be a major burden on our mental health, but there are strategies that can help you deal with it. Imagine you're in a stressful situation where you feel like you're losing control. An easy example of effective stress management could be consciously taking deep breaths. Take a moment to calm your thoughts and focus on your breath. This simple breathing exercise can help you regain inner peace and reduce stress levels.

Finding support:
It's important to know that you're not alone and can find support in difficult times. Often, we feel isolated and think that nobody can understand our feelings and challenges. But there are people willing to stand by us and support us. Imagine you're feeling overwhelmed and can't handle your mental health issues alone. An example of finding support could be confiding in someone. It could be a trusted friend, a family member, or a professional therapist. By opening up and talking about your feelings, you can gain understanding and valuable support to cope with your challenges.

Everyday examples:
To make the topic of dealing with mental health issues in everyday life even more tangible, we would like to present you with some specific examples that

aim to resonate with and encourage you. Imagine you've had a stressful day at work and feel exhausted.

An example of self-care could be consciously taking time for relaxation and rest. It could mean enjoying a warm bath, relaxing on the couch with a good book, or listening to your favorite music. By giving yourself these small breaks, you give your mind and body the opportunity to regenerate.

In terms of stress management, an example could be consciously taking a short break and doing a breathing exercise in stressful moments. Take a moment to take deep breaths and consciously release tension when exhaling. This simple method can help calm your thoughts and reduce stress.

"Final thoughts

Dealing with mental health issues in everyday life requires your active engagement and willingness to make changes. By taking care of yourself, applying effective stress management techniques, and seeking support, you can strengthen your mental health and lead a more fulfilling life. Let yourself be inspired and encouraged by the examples to find your own ways of dealing with your challenges. You are not alone on this journey, and together we can promote our mental health and achieve positive changes in our daily lives."

Chapter 15: Hope and Healing

Welcome to the final chapter of our book, which focuses on the topic of hope and healing. In this chapter, we want to present you with inspiring stories of people who have successfully overcome their mental health problems. We want to show you that healing is possible and that there is hope, even if you find yourself in a difficult situation right now. Take a moment to be touched and encouraged by the following stories.

Stories of courage and growth:

In this chapter, we want to introduce you to people who have gone through similar mental challenges as you. Success stories of individuals who have overcome depression, anxiety disorders, or other mental health issues.

Let's take the example of Lisa's story. She suffered from severe depression for many years and felt hopeless. However, with the support of her family, the professional help of a therapist, and her own determination, she managed to step out of the darkness step by step. Lisa shares how she was able to overcome her depression through self-belief and the willingness to make changes. Today, she lives a fulfilling life and serves as an inspiration to others struggling with similar issues.

Another case is the story of Michael. He battled anxiety disorders and social phobia for years, which greatly limited his life. But through a combination of psychotherapy, medication, and learning coping strategies, he gradually overcame his fears. Today, Michael is able to give public speeches and lead a fulfilling social life. His story shows that there are ways to manage anxieties and lead a fulfilling life, even when it initially seems hopeless.

Paths to healing:
In addition to these inspiring stories, we also want to present you with some proven paths to healing. There are various approaches that can help you cope with your mental health problems and strengthen your mental well-being. Psychotherapy is a widely used and effective method to address the roots of your issues and learn new coping strategies. Both cognitive-behavioral therapy and psychodynamic therapy have helped many people overcome their mental health problems.

In addition to therapy, medications can also play an important role. In some cases, a combination of psychotherapy and medication may be the best treatment option. However, it's important to note that each person is unique, and not every treatment method is suitable for everyone. Having an open conversation with a professional therapist or psychiatrist can help you find the right treatment option for your specific situation.

Hope and healing are not empty words but achievable goals. The stories of Lisa, Michael, and many others show that people are capable of overcoming their mental health problems and leading fulfilling lives. There may be times when you feel helpless and desperate, but remember that you are not alone.

There is support, professional help, and proven methods that can assist you on your path to healing.

Be open to change and accept the support offered to you. Believe in your own strengths and that you have the power to improve your situation. Every step you take, no matter how small, brings you closer to healing. Be patient with yourself and recognize that the path to healing may take time and effort.

"With this chapter, we want to encourage you and show you that there is hope even in the darkest moments. It is possible to overcome mental health problems and lead a fulfilling, happy life. Trust in your own strength and be open to the opportunities that come your way. You deserve healing and a life full of hope and satisfaction."

<u>Closing Words:</u>

With this book, "simple explanation of mental problems" we've tried to give you a comprehensible insight into the world of mental health and provide you with tools to promote your own mental well-being. We hope we've encouraged you to take a look within and pay attention to your own mental health.

We hope this book has sparked your interest and inspired you to explore more books and resources on this topic. The world of mental health is fascinating and offers a variety of approaches, techniques, and stories that can help you continue your journey to healing.

Invest in yourself and take time to care for your needs. Be open to new insights and ready to embrace change. With each step you take, you come closer to a life filled with well-being and inner strength.

We sincerely thank you for reading this book. It has been an honor to accompany you on your path to mental health. We hope you can apply the insights and tips in your daily life and that you're encouraged to continue taking care of your mental health.

Stay curious, stay strong, and be proud of the progress you've already made. Your mental health is invaluable and deserves your attention and care.

We wish you all the best on your journey to mental health and hope you continue to seek knowledge, support, and inspiring books.

Warm regards,

Kevin van Olafson